User Guide

Physical Examination and Health Assessment Online

for

Mosby's Guide to Physical Examination

Seventh Edition

By

Henry M. Seidel, MD
Professor Emeritus of Pediatrics
The Johns Hopkins University
School of Medicine
Baltimore, Maryland

Jane W. Ball, DrPH, RN, CPNP, DPNAP
Trauma Systems Consultant
American College of Surgeons
Gaithersburg, Maryland

Joyce E. Dains, DrPH, JD, RN, FNP-BC, DPNAP
Advanced Practice Nursing Program Director
The University of Texas
M. D. Anderson Cancer Center
Houston, Texas

John A. Flynn, MD, MBA
Clinical Director and Professor of Medicine
Division of General Internal Medicine
The Johns Hopkins University
School of Medicine
Baltimore, Maryland

Barry S. Solomon, MD, MPH
Assistant Professor of Pediatrics
Medical Director, Harriet Lane Clinic
Division of General Pediatrics and
Adolescent Medicine
The Johns Hopkins University
School of Medicine
Baltimore, Maryland

Rosalyn W. Stewart, MD, MS, MBA
Assistant Professor of Pediatrics and Medicine
Department of Internal Medicine and
Pediatrics
The Johns Hopkins University
School of Medicine
Baltimore, Maryland

Advanced Practice Case Studies by:

Diana Mertens, RN, CNM, MEd, DPH
Internship Coordinator
Graduate Nursing Program
School of Nursing and Health Services
Northern Illinois University
DeKalb, Illinois

Jason Underwood, MSEd
Department of Educational Technology
Research and Assessment
Northern Illinois University
DeKalb, Illinois

ELSEVIER
MOSBY

3251 Riverport Lane
Maryland Heights, Missouri 63043

PHYSICAL EXAMINATION AND HEALTH ASSESSMENT ONLINE FOR
MOSBY'S GUIDE TO PHYSICAL EXAMINATION
SEVENTH EDITION
Copyright © 2011 by Mosby, Inc., an affiliate of Elsevier Inc.

ISBN: 978-0-323-06542-9

Notices

Knowledge and best practice in this field are constantly changing. As new research and experience broaden our understanding, changes in research methods, professional practices, or medical treatment may become necessary.

Practitioners and researchers must always rely on their own experience and knowledge in evaluating and using any information, methods, compounds, or experiments described herein. In using such information or methods they should be mindful of their own safety and the safety of others, including parties for whom they have a professional responsibility.

With respect to any drug or pharmaceutical products identified, readers are advised to check the most current information provided (i) on procedures featured or (ii) by the manufacturer of each product to be administered, to verify the recommended dose or formula, the method and duration of administration, and contraindications. It is the responsibility of practitioners, relying on their own experience and knowledge of their patients, to make diagnoses, to determine dosages and the best treatment for each individual patient, and to take all appropriate safety precautions.

To the fullest extent of the law, neither the Publisher nor the authors, contributors, or editors, assume any liability for any injury and/or damage to persons or property as a matter of products liability, negligence or otherwise, or from any use or operation of any methods, products, instructions, or ideas contained in the material herein.

ISBN: 978-0-323-06542-9

Evolve® is a registered trademark of Elsevier Inc. in the United States and other jurisdictions.

Executive Editor: Robin Carter
Developmental Editor: Deanna Dedeke
Publishing Services Manager: Jeff Patterson
Book Production Project Manager: Tracey Schriefer
Associate eProject Manager: Kristin Zurliene

Printed in the United States of America

Last digit is the print number: 9 8 7 6 5 4 3

Working together to grow libraries in developing countries

www.elsevier.com | www.bookaid.org | www.sabre.org

ELSEVIER | BOOK AID International | Sabre Foundation

GETTING STARTED

If your course is being led by an instructor:

1. System

Your instructor will provide information about the system on which your course is being hosted. Evolve® courses can be run on a variety of systems and your instructor will decide which one is right for this course.

2. Username & Password

Your instructor will also provide you with the username and password needed to access the system where this course is located, or provide you with their Course ID to self-enroll.

3. Login & Enrollment Instructions

If your instructor's course is being hosted on the Evolve Learning System, please visit the **How To** section of the Evolve homepage at http://evolve.elsevier.com for detailed enrollment instructions. If your course is on a different system, your instructor will provide login information.

4. Access Code

The first time you access this course, you will need the access code located inside the front cover of this User Guide, regardless of which system is hosting the course. When you are prompted, enter the code **exactly** as it appears in this guide.

If you plan to take the course on your own:

(**Note:** By taking the course independently, you will not have any instructor to help you with the course. You will have 12 months from the date you are enrolled to complete the course.)

1. System

All independent learners are enrolled in a course hosted on the Evolve Learning System.

2. Login & Enrollment Instructions

For detailed enrollment instructions, please visit the **How To** section of the Evolve homepage at http://evolve.elsevier.com.

3. Username & Password

If you don't have an existing Evolve account, you will be able to create one during the self-enrollment process.

4. Access Code

The first time you access this course, you will need the access code located inside the front cover of this User Guide. When you are prompted, enter the code **exactly** as it appears in this guide.

SUPPORT INFORMATION

Visit the Evolve Support Portal at http://evolvesupport.elsevier.com to access the Evolve Knowledge Base, Downloads, and Support Ticket System. Live Evolve Support is also available 24/7 by calling 1-800-222-9570.

TECHNICAL REQUIREMENTS

To use an Evolve Online Course, you will need access to a computer that is connected to the Internet and equipped with web browser software that supports frames. For optimal performance, it is recommended that you have speakers and use a high-speed Internet connection. However, slower dial-up modems (56K minimum) are acceptable.

Screen Settings

For best results, the resolution of your computer monitor should be set at a minimum of 800 x 600. The number of colors displayed should be set to "thousands or higher" (High Color or 16 bit) or "millions of colors" (True Color or 24 bit). To set the resolution:

Windows
1. From the **Start** menu, select **Settings** and **Control Panel**.
2. Double-click on the **Display** icon.
3. Click on the **Settings** tab.
4. Under **Screen resolution** use the slider bar to select **800 by 600 pixels** (or greater).
5. In the **Colors** drop down menu, click on the arrow to show more settings.
6. Click on **High Color (16 bit)** or **True Color (24 bit)**.
7. Click on **Apply**.
8. Click on **OK**.
9. You may be asked to verify the setting changes. Click **Yes**.
10. You may be asked to restart your computer to accept the setting changes. Click **Yes**.

Macintosh
1. Select the **Monitors** control panel.
2. Select **800 x 600** (or greater) from the **Resolution** area.
3. Select **Thousands** or **Millions** from the **Colors** area.

Web Browsers

Supported web browsers include Microsoft Internet Explorer (IE) version 7.0 or higher and Mozilla Firefox version 3.0 or higher. The supported browser for Macs running OS X is Mozilla Firefox.

Whichever browser you use, the browser preferences must be set to enable cookies and the cache must be set to reload every time.

The most up-to-date information for browser settings can be found at http://windows.microsoft.com/en-us/windows/help for Internet Explorer and http://support.mozilla.com for Firefox.

Plug-Ins

Adobe Acrobat Reader

Download at: http://www.adobe.com

Apple QuickTime

Download at: http://www.apple.com

Adobe Flash Player

Download at: http://www.adobe.com

Adobe Shockwave Player

Download at: http://www.adobe.com

Microsoft Word Viewer

Download at: http://www.microsoft.com

Microsoft PowerPoint Viewer

Download at: http://www.microsoft.com

Enable Cookies

Browser	Steps
Internet Explorer (IE) 7.0 or higher	1. Select **Tools → Internet Options** on the menu bar. If you do not see the menu bar, hit the Alt key on your keyboard. 2. Select the **Privacy** tab. 3. Click the **Advanced** button. 4. Click the check box for **"Override Automatic Cookie Handling"**. 5. Click the radio button for **"Accept"** on both First & Third-party cookies. 6. Click the box for **"Always allow session cookies"**. 7. Click the **OK** button. 8. Click the **OK** button.
Mozilla Firefox 3.0 or higher	1. Select **Tools → Options** from the menu bar at the top. 2. Select the **Privacy** tab. 3. Assure that **"Use custom settings for history"** is selected in the drop-down menu. 4. Check the box for **"Accept Cookies from Sites"**. 5. Check the box for **"Accept third-party cookies"**. 6. Click the **OK** button.

Set Cache to Always Reload a Page

Browser	Steps
Internet Explorer (IE) 7.0 or higher	1. Select **Tools → Internet Options** on the menu bar. If you do not see the menu bar, hit the Alt key on your keyboard. 2. Select the **General** tab. 3. Click the button for **"Settings"** in the Browsing History section. 4. Click the radio button for **"Every time I visit the webpage"**. 5. Enter in **0** (or smallest number allowed) in the Disk space to Use section. 6. Click the **OK** button. 7. Click the **OK** button.